Intermittent Fasting for Women Over 50

The Complete Guide to Weight Loss, Increase Longevity and Balance Your Hormones

Joelle Coy

Table of Contents

Your free Gift!

Having purchased this book, you are entitled to an exclusive FREE gift!

You can have the **Audiobook** version for free just by signing up for a FREE 30-day trial on Audible!

FOLLOW STEPS BELOW TO GET STARTED!

1. Go to the page where you bought the book on Amazon

2. click on the audiobook version

3. Sign up and get your free copy NOW!

Introduction

Expectations are a powerful force! As people grow older, they almost welcome physical and mental deterioration. To some extent, wear and tear does happen to our bodies with time because we are using it at full capacity each day. But much of the decline in stamina is a direct result of our own minds. Society perceives older adults as weak, fragile, and "on their way out." Seniors themselves come to accept these perceptions and expect their bodies to start showing signs of decline such as bone density loss, lower muscle mass, high or low blood pressure, slower metabolism, accumulated body fat, problems with blood sugar tolerance, achy joints, and so on. The strength of the mind can wield a lot of power over the body!

These self-limiting beliefs make people take measures that can be detrimental to their health or ignore it thinking it will improve on its own. For example, if you believe that as one grows older, it is inevitable to lose muscle mass, accumulate fat around the waist, discover more wrinkles, ridges or spots on the skin, and other flaws linked to getting old, you are unlikely to engage in healthy habits to fix them. But once a person can change their perception of aging, they will have the motivation to take deliberate keeping their body in sound health for the rest of their life. One such action is fasting.

It is common for women approaching their golden age to harbor a secret fear of losing the vitality and beauty that comes with youth. Some women want to avoid this time like the plague because of concerns about not being able to remain strong, sexy, and attractive. But all that fear is unnecessary because it's possible to retain strength, intelligence, soft and tender skin, vibrancy, and all the important qualities of a healthy woman as long as she engages in the right habits. By implementing these suggestions and recommendations, you will begin to fall in love with this special time in life.

Coming of age is not synonymous with inability, and this book will prove that to you! But beyond superficial proof, you will be learning new healthy eating habits to make you look and feel younger than your biological age. Weight loss may seem like the only proclaimed benefit of intermittent fasting, but you will discover that there are advantages to a proper diet that go beyond weight loss.

Your overall health and wellbeing aren't just affected by what you eat, but when you eat. Right now you might be thinking it's pointless to start a new eating habit as an older adult. These thoughts are what put your health in a perpetual state of decline plus it's never too late, especially for something that will improve your quality of life.

Intermittent fasting is quickly becoming the "it" thing for people of different age ranges. Many, especially young adults, are frothing over the idea of a new, quick, cost effective way to lose weight and are eager to try it for themselves. This mentality is driven by the need to stay current or remain "on brand" with their social media presence. The downside is that people get on a trend without doing their homework to retain the proper knowledge and risk involved. This book overrides the fad mentality and will present you with unbiased information about intermittent fasting, especially as it relates to women over 50. I have removed unnecessary information that is irrelevant to those outside this age range so that older adults can have something to relate to.

Getting older is a wonderful experience every woman should look forward to, and celebrated as not everyone has the option. It is my sincere hope that after reading these pages, you will find the motivation to apply what you have learned and reap the numerous benefits of controlling your diet.

Chapter 1:
Intermittent Fasting –
The Basics

For many, fasting has a bad reputation, with religious connotations surrounding it as a form of penance or self-punishment for wrongdoing. To others, the idea of going without food is considered unrealistic and extremely unsafe. But all these notions are deeply rooted in misconceptions and unfounded fears of starvation or guilt over those around the world who actually can't afford food. Eating is how the body survives, but is not designed to eat every few hours as our normal behavior suggests. Filling your body with food 3 to 6 times every day actually has the ability to diminish your overall physical, mental, and emotional health as you age.

From an evolutionary perspective, early primitive humans went without food for significant amounts of time and as a result were seemingly healthier, stronger, and leaner than our modern day selves. Several scientific studies have shown the immense benefits associated with fasting. Some of these benefits, just to name a few, include weight loss, treatment for obesity, and even improvements to symptoms of Alzheimer's. But you do not need a pre-existing medical condition to practice fasting. Early humans went without food as a necessary part of life, not because they were trying to improve a condition. Before you decide to start fasting, you need to determine what it entails and whether or not it is suitable for you.

What Is Intermittent Fasting?

Intermittent fasting is a practice of abstaining from food for an extended amount of time. It is a pattern of eating that increases your fasted state while decreasing your fed state. But simply abstaining from food doesn't mean you are fasting. Starvation, for example, is not fasting. A person who starves, wants food but has no options to eat and can result in nutrient deprivation. Also, a person who eats nothing after dinner say around 8 pm, for example, until the next morning, may have gone without food for 12 hours, but that doesn't translate to fasting.

The person who eats nothing else after dinner until the next morning may choose to stay away from food for that time but if the hunger becomes too much they might have a quick snack at midnight. It happens, hunger isn't a great feeling. Also, they might have meals at varying, random times without keeping to any schedule. Or they don't know what they are doing or even that they are fasting, so there is no purposefulness in the act. For abstinence from food to be considered intermittent fasting, it has to be a conscious choice, followed on a schedule, and done with a purpose. Whether the goal is to treat a condition or just maintain sound health, a target will keep you on track with your eating plan.

Intermittent fasting follows a schedule – a preplanned, stretch of time when you completely abstain from eating food (the fasting window) and a shorter period known as the eating window. There are quite a few different intermittent schedules or regimens that have been created that produce slightly different results. Whichever one you choose to follow is entirely up to you, but the important thing is to be consistent in developing a plan.

You may not be eating, but it should never stop you from drinking water. It may seem like a no brainer but it's important to remind you that water intake during fasting is a requirement to stay alive, and stay healthy. You can drink other liquids such as unsweetened coffee, tea, and other liquids that do not contain calories in the fasting hours to break up the monotony or curb any cravings. It can be tough for anyone, and have more specific effects on women in particular. To give you a better idea, here's a brief science of how intermittent fasting works.

How It Works

When you eat, your food is converted into sugar that serves as your body's fuel and is stored in the liver. As you eat, your insulin levels increase to help the body store this influx of energy. However, your liver can only store so much, and it is a limited amount, before it reaches capacity. Your body fat serves as this backup storage so when your liver is full, the excess energy is stored as body fat. Although energy stored in the liver is accessible, body fat has unlimited storage capacity.

Eating gives your body a lot of work to do – breaking down food particles, digesting, and extracting energy and nutrients. The periods when you are not eating, your body turns to the stored energy to fuel your activities and keep you going.

What this means is that when you are fasting, there is a significant absence of energy coming from meals. Within hours, energy from your liver is depleted, and your insulin level drops. Your body senses this change and turns to the backup storage to begin using stored energy in the form of body fat. In other words, fasting helps your body burn fat. Essentially, you are either accumulating energy by eating or burning up energy when you are not. The key to maintaining a healthy weight and generally staying healthy is to strike a balance between storing and using energy.

Your body does not need you to feed it frequently for it to have enough energy. If you are a normal healthy person, your body already has enough energy to last you longer than you realize. If you don't give your body time to use its stored energy, it can result in being overweight. The reason for storing energy in the first place is so that it can be used later. How can it be used if you don't allow your body a break from accumulating it? If you were meant to eat continuously, there would be no need for anything in place to reserve it.

On the other hand, staying away from food for too long can have adverse effects on your body. As much as you don't want to be overweight, being underweight is never healthy, and why you need to find a balance between eating and not eating. A good way to do that is by introducing a pattern of eating that helps you to reduce the number of hours you eat (without necessarily focusing on reducing calories). When you reduce your eating hours, your calorie intake declines.

Benefits of Intermittent Fasting

The benefit of intermittent fasting, especially for middle-aged and older women, is discussed throughout this book and here is a quick summary of the benefits that come from the practice.

1. Builds mental and physical resilience.
2. Improves memory.
3. Boosts overall energy.
4. Promotes cellular repairs.
5. Significantly minimizes insulin resistance by reducing blood sugar levels.
6. Increases the body's resistance to diseases as a result of increased cell stress response rate.
7. Improves sleep patterns.
8. Reduces cholesterol levels.
9. Increases lean muscle.
10. Decreases cravings for sugars (carbohydrates).
11. Possibility of reversing type 2 diabetes.
12. Significantly reduces bloating and decreases inflammation.
13. Improves digestion and gut health.
14. Boosts growth hormones.
15. It helps you live longer.
16. Significantly improves the body's ability to burn fat.

A good way to get the benefits of intermittent fasting is to approach it as a lifestyle change instead of a band-aid remedy for long-term problems. This means you are not in a hurry to make drastic changes to your eating pattern and won't risk pushing yourself unnecessarily. Approach intermittent fasting as a gradual way of detoxifying your body, and your cells will get to work ridding your insides of free radicals and fixing broken cells. Now you might be asking if intermittent fasting is safe for middle-aged and older women?

Who Should Fast?

Regardless of the many benefits of intermittent fasting, the practice is not suitable for everyone. Keep in mind that this practice is supposed to improve your overall health and fitness level and not to create more health problemsIf you have any of the conditions listed below, intermittent fasting may not be suitable for you.

1. Chronic stress and diseases.
2. Eating disorders (anorexia or bulimia).
3. Malnourishment.
4. Sleep disorders (deprivation or insomnia).
5. Others are pregnant women or breastfeeding mothers.

You may require medical supervision while fasting if you have diabetes, are on any form of medication, or have painful swelling in your joints caused by excess deposits of uric acid. However, this condition is more prevalent in men more so than in women. From this list you will see nothing suggests intermittent fasting is unsafe for older adults or specifically women over. The notion that intermittent fasting is not safe for older adults can be linked to a general misconception of the term 'stress.' While it is true that excessive stress is not safe for older adults or anyone for that matter, it is good to highlight that there is negative and positive stress. Positive stress (eustress) varies from from negative (distress) and is crucial for survival.

When exposed to stress in small doses, it has the ability to motivate you to face daily challenges and reach your goals with a certain amount of power behind it. Small doses of stress can boost memory retention and sharpen focus. Intermittent fasting, when done correctly (for short periods), is a positive stressor that benefits the body and mind. In fact, a study from a group of scientists from the University of Florida found that fasting can make your cells more resilient to stress (Douglas, et. al., 2015).

One good way to check if you are correctly fasting correctly and is a positive source of stress is to ask yourself, *"Do I feel excited about fasting? Is it something I want to do or something I have to do?"* For the practice to be sustainable, you need to approach it as something you want or choose to do because you are eager. If it feels like you're being forced, you're adding undue stress to an already stress-inducing activity.

Chapter 2:
Types of Intermittent Fasting

Now that you have a better understanding of intermittent fasting and what it's all about, it is time to consider the common types of fasting schedules or regimens available to you. As you go through this chapter, you may find one or two fasting approaches appealing, but before you start, try the example at the end of this chapter first.

Intermittent Fasting Regimen

16:8 Regimen

This is one of the more popular types of intermittent fasting. The schedule is straightforward and relatively easy to do. It involves eating all your meals within an 8-hour window and staying away from food (including snacks) except water and calorie-free beverages for a 16-hour fasting window. This is a safe option, and you can do it daily or five days a week for an extended period. Here's a typical example:

For the next three months, you would opt to eat two or three meals daily between 11 am and 7 pm on Mondays, Tuesdays, Wednesdays. Eat normally on

Thursdays and continue the fasting pattern on Fridays and Saturdays. Eat normally on Sundays and repeat the eating pattern for the next seven days until the three months are over.

However, since the best way to approach intermittent fasting is to make it a lifestyle change, try to implement it four days a week, at the most. That way, you can make it into a habit and keep up with it.

The Crescendo Method

This method of intermittent fasting is a great way to help your body get used to fasting without any major disturbance to sensitive hormones. The schedule is flexible and allows your body to have adequate rest.

The crescendo fasting schedule, as the name implies, involves a gradual increase in the hours you are required to fast usually not more than 12 to 16 hours for a couple of days in a week. Here's an example of how to use the crescendo fasting schedule. Fast for 12 hours on day 1. On day 2, increase the fasting period to 13 hours. And on day 3, add two extra hours to the fasting window to make it 15 hours. From day 4 to day 7, eat normally. The next week, you can repeat the same thing with a slight change in day 3 to bring the hours to 16. The eating window for this type of regimen is anywhere between 8 and 12 hours. It is a safe way to fast, requiring a schedule and a lot of dedication.

20:4 Regimen

In this fasting regimen, all your meals are consumed within 4 hours, and then you are required to stay away from food for 20 straight hours. Reading that sentence may have you shaking your head, because sure that number is big and can seem impossible not eating for an entire day. Consider this though, that 20 hours includes the 6 to 8 hours of sleeping time required, so you're really only awake for 12 hours of the fast. For example: you eat your meals between 2 and 6 pm, then fast until 2 pm the next day. And from 10 pm or whenever your bedtime might be, you will sleep until 5 am or so, leaving only about 8 hours before your next meal.

You may choose to eat one big meal or two smaller meals within the 4-hour eating window. The important thing is to focus on eating unprocessed and organic foods and avoid any junk food such as candy, fast or fried foods, refined carbohydrates, chips, pretzels, cookies, donuts, soda, and fruit juice, etc.

Practice this fasting regimen in moderation. Do not engage in it for more than a couple of weeks, especially if you are a beginner. Also, remember to skip a day or two on this regimen. Continuing this fast consecutively can leave you feeling very weak and foggy. It is easy to confuse the 20:4 intermittent fasting with a similar eating plan known as the Warrior Diet. Although the Warrior Diet uses the same 20:4 fasting and eating windows, it is technically not the same as intermittent fasting.

The Warrior Diet is designed to mimic the eating patterns of early humans who didn't eat three or more meals a day. It is also an attempt to replicate the eating pattern of ancient fighters who ate very little during the day and feasted at night, hence the name. However, this meal plan allows you to eat small amounts of fruits and vegetables, eggs, and dairy in addition to tea, black coffee, and water during the 20-hour fasting window. After the window, you can eat anything you want for the four hours. Nevertheless, eating clean is still encouraged. There is a 3-week eating plan to help practitioners get used to the diet before diving in.

24-Hour Regimen (aka Eat-Stop-Eat)

The 24-hour fasting schedule or Eat-Stop-Eat is a One Meal A Day (OMAD) regimen. The regimen allows you to eat only once in 24 hours. For example, if you eat at 4 pm on day 1, you are expected to eat nothing except water and calorie-free beverages until 4 pm on day 2. Although you eat daily on this schedule, you are doing so only once in a complete 24-hour cycle. If you use this method for weight loss, it is important to eat normally when you break your fast. That is to say, eat the usual amount of food you would have if you were not fasting. Never attempt to restrict calories when doing this.

Since all your foods are consumed at once, the eating window for this type of fast is zero. Moderation is the watchword when using this regimen. It is not advised to use this method continuously or on consecutive days. Before using this regimen, practice with a 14 or 16-hour fasting window and gradually increase your fasting hours until you can last 24 hours without food.

The Alternate-Days Regimen

This regimen involves going without food for an entire day and then eating the next day freely. This means that you are only consuming half of the food you would normally eat and automatically reducing your calorie intake in the process. On fasting days, water and calorie-free beverages are allowed. If you choose to go this route, only try it twice a week to give your body enough time to recover from the rigors of fasting.

5:2 Diet "Fasting"

Technically, this is more of a diet plan than a fasting regimen. However, many people find it easy to start with the 5:2 Diet before going fully into intermittent fasting. Typically, it involves eating as you normally would for five days and then "fasting" for two days. The "fasting" in this sense means restricting your calorie consumption. On fasting days, you are required to restrict your calorie intake to only 500 calories. You can consume the entire 500 calories in one meal or spread them throughout your meals for each of the two fasting days.

For example, you can eat normal on Monday and limit your calorie consumption to only 500 on Tuesday. Eat normal on Wednesday and Thursday, and then "fast" on Friday. Eat normal for the rest of the week and then repeat the same pattern the following week.

Others

Other extended fasting regimens last for 36, 48, and 72 hours. The human body can survive a long time without food. But it is not necessary to go to such an extreme route to appease vanity or achieve anything superficial. You can cause severe health issues if you engage in such practices for a silly reason and do not advise women to engage in such extended fasts, no matter their age.

Safety Tips for Practicing Intermittent Fasting

Intermittent fasting can trigger hormonal changes that impact your entire internal system. Your body functions such as blood pressure regulation, metabolism, digestion, and energy production, are controlled by interconnected hormones. Introducing any major change that affects one hormone can cause a ripple effect on the others. This is why before you begin to put your body through the stress of going without food for longer than you're used to, it is crucial to understand how to do so safely.

Keep the following safety tips in mind as you select a fasting regimen to practice.

1. As an older adult who is getting into intermittent fasting for the first time, aim to fast between 12 and 16 hours a day. Going without food for longer than that may put unnecessary strain on your body. Remember that you have spent more than half a decade training your body to expect food at certain intervals. Staying away from food too long may cause unpleasant side effects that will defeat the goal of intermittent fasting.

2. Begin your fasting regimen by delaying your normal eating time by one or two extra hours. Within those extra hours, try not to snack. Instead, drink water if you feel hungry. The example at the end of this chapter will illuminate this.

3. In the first three weeks or thereabout of beginning this new eating pattern, it is better to not fast on consecutive days. Give an interval of one or two days between fasting days. For example, if you choose to fast for 16 hours a day, you could do that on Monday, Wednesday, and Friday. Even if your goal is rapid weight loss, avoid fasting for seven straight days, especially as a beginner. Your body needs to rest from the stress brought on by your new practice. Do not let the obsession with weight loss obscure your better judgment.

4. Once you are able to fast for longer than 16 hours, I strongly suggest not exceeding 24 hours. A prolonged period of fasting can result in harmful effects, including irritability, dehydration, fainting, mood changes, feeling very weak (lack of energy), and difficulty in focusing. To avoid these negative effects, stick to fasting for shorter periods, particularly if you are new to the practice.

5. Discontinue your fast if at any time you start to feel unwell. It is normal to feel hungry, irritable, or a bit tired, but feeling unwell is a red flag. If you have reasons to be concerned during fasting, it is advisable to stop at once, eat something small and seek medical attention.

What to Do If Intermittent Fasting Isn't Safe for You

As much as intermittent fasting itself is a safe practice, it's possible it might not be suitable for you. What can you do if this is the case? Should you have a poor diet and lifestyle because it tastes really good and just easier? Of course, not. Fasting might not be for you but healthy nutrition is what every human on this planet should strive for. Try to limit your intake of heavily processed foods as much as you can and make a conscious effort to eat only whole foods. Also, if it is medically advised, you should already be committed to following a light to medium workout routine.

Never push your body to do something that could be deemed medically unsafe. As a woman with several years of experience, you know the dangers of joining in fads when it is not in your best interest. For most men, intermittent fasting may come easier, with less problems as it doesn't impact their hormones the same way. But for women, this practice can take a huge toll on them whether they are at the reproductive age, menopausal stage, or postmenopausal age. Remember that whatever can negatively impact your reproductive hormones when you are at a childbearing age, can also trigger unpleasant reactions in your system even when you have passed the childbearing age.

It is important to realize that there are other ways you can remain healthy without jeopardizing your overall well being. While I suggest that every woman try intermittent fasting, never put your health at risk even if someone tells you it's a miracle cure.

An Example of Easing Into Fasting Regimens

Here is a 5-day fasting plan that illustrates how you can ease into intermittent fasting. I have used the 16:8 method in this example. Whichever fasting regimen you decide to follow, it is important to start gradually.

Day 1: Stop eating after dinner

- Enjoy your meals until dinner, after which you should stop eating any other food. For example, if you have dinner by 8 pm, you should not consume any other food after that until the next day. This may sound easy until you find yourself reaching for a quick snack while lounging on the couch watching tv. No food means no crackers, cookies or popcorn! Instead, reach for a glass of water to curb hunger.

Day 2: Delay breakfast

- When you wake up on day 2, hold off a bit on breakfast. Don't skip it but delay it a little. By 8 am, you have successfully fasted for 12 hours straight! Wasn't that easy?
- While you are delaying breakfast, drink water, black coffee, or unsweetened tea.
- Keep yourself busy until 11 am and then have breakfast. You have fasted for 15 hours!
- Since you won't likely feel hungry right away, you can delay lunch till 3 pm.
- Repeat dinner at 8 pm and follow the no-eating rule until the next day.

Day 3: Rinse and Repeat!

- As before, delay breakfast until 11 am to give you a 15 hour fast.

- Make sure not to snack between breakfast and lunch by 3 pm. If you feel hungry, drink water, or any calorie-free drink.
- Eat dinner at 8 pm, and say goodbye to food until the next day.

Day 4: Add an Extra Hour to Your Fasting Window

- Instead of eating at 11 am, delay your first meal for the day until noon. You are only adding an extra hour, so there should be no difficulty there. And just in case you didn't notice, you have successfully fasted for 16 hours straight!
- Keep your energy up and the feeling of hunger down by drinking water and other non-calorie drinks any time you get the urge to eat something or you feel hungry.
- Remember to stop eating after 8 pm.

Day 5: Reinforce Your New Eating Habit

- Commit to following this pattern of eating for a couple of days each week for the determined time. Write down how the new eating pattern affects your overall health and well being and make adjustments where necessary.

Remember to adjust the hours and timing to suit your preferred fasting regimen.

Chapter 3:
Fasting and the Female Body

A woman's body is a delicate creation! While a man can engage in many stress-inducing activities (such as extended fasting, extreme dieting, and intense workouts) without any significant effects on their body, females aren't designed to handle such high amounts of stressful impact, and for a good reason. The female body is designed to house another human to ensure the continuation of the human race. Whether or not a woman chooses to get pregnant and give birth during her childbearing years, it doesn't change her chemical composition. She is still a woman with very sensitive hormones. What impact does it have on the female hormones, especially for women over 50?

Your Hormones at 50+ Years

One of the major health concerns for women over 50 is menopause. Luckily these major hormonal changes leading to menopause don't just happen overnight, it takes anywhere from 3 to 15 years for these changes to happen, make an impact, and for hormones to become relatively stable. That's a long time to endure these unpleasant feelings. On average, women experience menopause at age 51, but it can occur as early as the 30s in some women and as late as the 60 for others (Stoppler, 2019).

At the onset of menopause, when your chemical messengers are unstable, it is not uncommon to wake up some mornings and feel as if you've just run a marathon on crutches. Your hormones can fluctuate dramatically and cause you to become sensitive like never before The initial symptoms such as hot flashes, night sweats, dry skin, hair loss, tender and small breasts, insomnia, vaginal dryness, low sex drive, andof course, mood swings are indications of perimenopause.

The female sex hormones (estrogen and progesterone) are unstable during this period. In some postmenopausal women, testosterone levels become higher than estrogen and progesterone levels and can result in insulin resistance, higher triglycerides (too much fat in the body that can lead to heart attack, stroke, and heart diseases), and a higher risk of developing breast cancer (Yasui, et al., 2012).

When you've gone a full 12 months without menstruation, most of these early symptoms will subside. Some will even disappear altogether because, at that stage, your hormones have stabilized or are in steady decline. But there's still one major problem: weight gain. It is normal to put on some weight during perimenopause and menopause. A little extra padding can even be beneficial at this stage of life. The fat tissues can be your body's extra if you get sick and as estrogen gets down-regulated by your ovaries, your fatty tissues step in to up-regulate.

However, when your estrogen levels become too high in relation to your progesterone levels, it can result in significant weight gain, especially in the waistline or on the hips. To achieve a healthy weight at this stage of your life, you will need to be deliberate about maintaining the balance between these hormones. Besides the sex hormones estrogen, progesterone, and testosterone, let's briefly look at how other hormones that control your weight (with particular attention on insulin) can be effectively managed.

Insulin Resistance

Weight gain has been linked to insulin resistance in postmenopausal women. Except for the obese, insulin resistance seems to play a role in weight gain for many postmenopausal women, especially those with lower BMI (Howard, et. al, 2004). But what exactly is insulin resistance? What are its causes, and how can you prevent or manage it?

Think of the hormones in your body as command centers that deliver instructions to your cells. The hormone insulin instructs them to extract sugar (glucose) required for body fuel from your blood. In a healthy person, the cells receive this instruction and promptly comply. But when the cells begin to ignore the insulin command center – specifically the cells in the muscles, body fat, and liver – the person is labeled as insulin resistant. Their cells are no longer responding to the instructions from insulin to extract glucose from the blood. This refusal to comply with instructions from the hormone insulin means that your body no longer has unfettered access to its fuel (glucose) and can't function optimally.

Although your body fights courageously to defeat these disobedient or resistant cells by producing more insulin, the battle cannot go on indefinitely. After a while, the cells of your pancreas will grow tired of producing more and more insulin. Soon, your pancreas will throw in the towel. If this happens, it won't be long before excess glucose accumulates in your blood since it is not being extracted and used for fuel. Excess blood sugar levels can result in Non-Alcoholic Fatty Liver Disease (NAFLD) – a precursor to liver damage and heart disease. Also, too much glucose in your blood can increase the risk of developing prediabetes and type 2 diabetes (American Journal of Managed Care, 2013).

Factors such as smoking and being overweight (obesity) can lead to insulin resistance. Other factors include age, excess fat, especially in the belly region, a sedentary lifestyle, and poor sleeping habits, particularly sleep deprivation.

Symptoms of Insulin Resistance

Metabolic syndrome. If at any time, you begin to have any three of the following symptoms, it is a strong indication that your body is resisting naturally produced insulin:

- High triglycerides: Triglycerides are a type of fat found in your blood. When triglycerides levels become equal or greater than 150 mg/dL, it is likely to increase the hardening of the arteries. There is a higher risk of heart attack, stroke, and other heart diseases if that happens.
- High fasting blood sugar: Blood sugar or glucose levels are usually slightly higher in the mornings, that's why it is called fasting blood sugar. Healthy blood sugar levels are usually between 80 – 130 mg/dL before meals and below 180 mg/dL about two hours after eating. But when fasting blood

sugar exceeds the normal levels, it could be an indication of a metabolic syndrome.

- High blood sugar: Also known as hyperglycemia, high blood sugar refers to elevated levels of glucose in the blood. It can cause frequent urination, frequent feeling of thirst, and a higher volume of glucose in the urine. Blood sugar level is said to be high when it is above 130 mg/dL before eating or above 180 mg/dL after eating.
- High blood pressure: A blood pressure higher than 130/85 mmHg is indicative of a metabolic syndrome.
- Low high-density lipoprotein levels (HDLs): HDL cholesterol, also called the good cholesterol, helps your body to get rid of other forms of harmful cholesterol from your system. An ideal HDL level is 60 mg/dL and above. A level less than 40 mg/dL is not healthy.

Excess fat on your waistline. If your waist area is beginning to show signs of accumulated fat, it might be an indication that you are developing insulin resistance. And if unexplainable dark patches begin to show up on your skin, particularly behind your neck, groin, or armpit, it could be an indicator. Usually, this only occurs in severe cases of insulin resistance and is known as acanthosis nigricans.

Preventive Measures

The good news is that it is possible to prevent and even reverse insulin resistance, especially at its onset. As a woman who is already in her golden years, it is in your best interest to engage in some (or all) of these practices as much as possible. Good health, staying fit and strong, and enjoying longevity doesn't happen by accident. It requires conscious or deliberate actions.

Get involved in weight loss programs! While many diet programs may lead to weight loss, some of them can be too demanding and restrictive. Sustaining weight loss may not be feasible if the method for achieving it is too tasking. A better alternative to help keep your weight healthy is intermittent fasting, especially if you make a lifestyle change rather than a rapid weight loss attempt. As you grow older, you must allow your body enough time to digest and use up enough energy from your meals before shoving down another meal. One of the more apparent benefits of intermittent fasting is weight loss. If you can maintain a healthy weight as you age, your chances of developing insulin resistance (and all its attendant problems) grow slimmer.

Getting older is not an excuse for living a non-active lifestyle. To enjoy your advanced years, a regimented exercise program should be a central part of your lifestyle. The good thing about working out is that you are not limited to just a gym membership. In the next chapter, you will learn some simple but effective exercises you can perform at home with small equipment. For a woman above 50, the key to getting impressive results with exercises is not how difficult or tedious the workout routine is or the length of the workout. The key to success with exercise is consistency even if it is a low-impact exercise, which I highly recommend. Performing exercises at least 30 minutes a day can greatly reduce your risk of developing insulin resistance.

Rest and quality sleep are also a big part of healthy living. It is not necessarily true that sleep declines as a person grows older. You still need between 7 and 8 hours of restful sleep even as you grow older. Without adequate sleep, your chances of developing high blood sugar levels increases. To give you an idea, scientists say that one sleepless night and an entire six months of a high-fat diet can mess with insulin sensitivity at almost the same rate (Science Daily, 2015).

Other Important Hormones That Can Impact Your Weight

<u>Cortisol - The Stress Hormone</u>

When your body senses stress, your adrenal glands release the hormone cortisol to help you deal with the stress. However, if you put your body through continued stress such as prolonged fasting or stringent diets over a long period, it can lead to a chronically elevated level of cortisol which is a situation you don't want to find yourself in. This situation can cause overeating and significant weight gain. One study showed that women who followed a low-calorie diet had increased cortisol levels and also felt more stressed than their counterparts on a normal diet (Tomiyama, et. al., 2010). To reduce cortisol levels, and by extension, adverse response to stress, engage in activities that soothe you, such as uninterrupted sleep, spending time with loved ones, and meditation. During your fasting window, it is a good practice to create time to meditate or at least listen to soothing music as this can decrease cortisol levels.

<u>Leptin - The Satiety Hormone</u>

Leptin is produced mainly in your fat cells. When you eat, leptin tells your brain when you have had enough. This instruction makes you think it's time to stop eating. But instead of high levels of leptin in the body to reduce your appetite, it works the other way round. The higher your leptin, the more you will eat. This is an indication of resistance and works similar to insulin resistance. Too much leptin means that your brain is not receiving the 'you are full' instruction. So your brain assumes you are still hungry even if you are overeating and have more than enough energy in storage.

Weight loss can help you maintain a normal leptin level. Getting adequate body movement through exercise, in addition to quality sleep, can help to boost your leptin sensitivity. By including fatty fish and more of other anti-inflammatory foods in your meals can help improve leptin sensitivity. Avoid excessive calorie restriction as this can deprive your body of vital nutrients and disrupt the production of hormones. Once your hormones are disrupted, it can lead to slower metabolism as well as mess with leptin levels.

Ghrelin - The Hunger Hormone

Ghrelin is triggered when your stomach is empty. It tells your brain that you need to eat, and makes you start feeling hungry. Usually, your ghrelin level is at its peak when you are hungry and drops significantly after your meal. But in obese people, ghrelin levels only decrease slightly after meals. This means that their brains aren't flagged to stop and they often end up consuming too much.

A good way to deal with this hormone problem is to limit or avoid sugar-sweetened drinks as they can weaken your ghrelin response after a meal. Having adequate protein in your meals can also help. This is why it is best to eat clean when you fast intermittently. You're doing your health goals any favors by fasting for long hours only to eat junk when it really needs nutrients and vitamins.

<u>Neuropeptide Y (NPY) - The Appetite Hormone</u>

The Neuropeptide Y hormone is produced by brain cells and those in the nervous system. It stimulates appetite, especially those pesky cravings for carbohydrates that never seem to be satiated. The hormone is highest when you go without food, as done with fasting. Elevated levels of NPY can result in overeating and abdominal fat gain. An effective way to maintain healthy levels of NPY is to avoid fasting for too long. Engaging in prolonged fasting (over 24 hours) can significantly increase NPY levels.

Age-Related Issues

For many postmenopausal women – mostly women in their late 60s and early 70s – the issue is not so much about weight gain as it is about frailness, risk of chronic diseases, a lack of vigor, and a host of other factors that can cut short longevity and put their health on a downward spiral.

Medications may offer temporary relief, but are the unpleasant side effects worth it? Are women doomed to a life of discomfort, soreness, irritation, and an inevitable decline in vitality as they age? For many women who can't seem to see a satisfactory solution, the future appears dark and full of anxiety. This notion may be largely responsible for why some women dread growing old. They obsess unnecessarily with staying young and would put their bodies through unnecessarily complicated diets just to remain healthy and strong as they age. Unfortunately, a lot of women give up on stringent diets and other difficult lifestyle changes that promise vitality and longevity.

As a woman, you can age gracefully without medications or following some exacting lifestyle changes. All you need is modifying your eating pattern as introduced in Chapter 1. But before you start making changes to the timing of your meals, it is important to heed the series of suggestions already given in this chapter to avoid possible negative impacts on your system. Even women of childbearing age can be negatively impacted by fasting because anything affecting a woman's reproductive hormones can certainly impact her overall health and wellbeing. And although most women over 50 are generally not looking to have kids, fasting can still disrupt body function.

Intermittent Fasting for Women Over 50

Intermittent fasting is not only safe but it is a very healthy practice for women over 50. Middle-aged and older women can gain a lot more than weight loss from fasting intermittently. In fact, the impact of intermittent fasting on cellular health is a key strategy for longevity, especially for older women.

When you stay away from food for longer periods than your body is used to, you allow your cells to carry out their natural function of detoxifying and cleaning themselves. During the series of metabolic activities that take place in your body, a lot of accumulated debris is left behind. Fasting helps to get rid of the debris and cause regeneration. A kind of reset.

As mentioned before, positive stressors are what you want. Intermittent fasting induces positive stress in a similar way exercises do to the body. By breaking down and rebuilding muscles, exercises make your muscles stronger and resilient. In the same way, staying away from food for longer than usual periods can put positive stressors on your body and help in the following ways:

1. **Resets circadian rhythms**: The circadian rhythm is your internal clock that regulates almost every bodily process. Negative stress can disrupt the internal clock and lead to a host of negative effects, including sleep disorders. One common cause of circadian rhythm disruption is menopause. But menopausal and postmenopausal women who practice intermittent fasting can enjoy the benefit of a regular-functioning internal clock.

2. **Improves heart function**: The heart cells can require high energy to function properly. Besides carbs, fat, and amino acids, the energy needs of your heart cells can be supplied through ketones activated by fasting. Ketones help to optimize your heart's performance. It can also protect your heart from injury and inflammation.

3. **Reboots your gut flora**: Intermittent fasting helps your gut health and your digestive system to reboot. This reset should happen regularly as the health of your digestive system determines the performance of your immune system. Also, your mood and mental health are connected to the health of your gut flora.

4. **Improves brain function**: When you fast, ketones are produced to fuel your brain. Ketones generate fewer injurious

reactive oxygen species (ROS). This means your brain performs better when it is powered by ketones instead of glucose.

Intermittent fasting, when practiced correctly, can act as maintenance of your body's various systems. Keep in mind that intermittent fasting is a pattern of eating, not stop and start eating. It is incomplete without proper re-feeding. Many of the "miracles" of fasting actually take place during the period of reintroducing food after cellular cleansing during the fasting period. So don't deprive yourself of healthy and normal-sized meals after fasting and remember to give up snacking, especially after dinner. To make your systems harmonize, you must synchronize. Nights are meant for sleeping, and your circadian system is cued for that. If you snack after dinner, it can throw your circadian system out of sync and mess with your natural ability to repair.

Listen to Your Body

As a woman over 50, you don't need to try very hard to know what your body is telling you. The advice to *pay attention to your body*, is necessary for younger women in particular because some of them may not treat their body the best or know what their hormones are signaling. By the time a woman gets to 50, she is well aware of how her body communicates.

Nevertheless, it is possible to assume that what works for one healthy woman is also working for others in her age group and on the same health level. As much as it is important to engage in practices that keep you healthy, you need to pay attention to how you feel inside because that is how your hormones tell you what is working for you. Keep tabs on hormonal health because that is one of the greatest risks women of all ages face when they fast. It is not just estrogen and other sex hormones that are important. Your thyroid, cortisol, and follicle-stimulating hormones (FSH) all need to be at equilibrium or near-perfect balance as much as possible.

Your hormones may respond negatively to excessive stress that can be caused by combining intermittent fasting with dieting. It doesn't matter if you know someone who successfully combined fasting and dieting. What matters is what your body tells you. Staying fit and healthy should be fun and not feel like punishment. As a woman in her golden years, if you have decided to try intermittent fasting, I suggest that you focus only on intermittent fasting to the exclusion of dieting.

Chapter 4:
Intermittent Fasting
and Exercise

Many people will ask if it is safe to combine fasting with exercise. I am here to say it is. However, some factors need to be considered before combining the two. First, the type of fasting regimen should be considered alongside the physical, mental, and psychological health of the individual. Women with existing medical conditions should not combine fasting with exercises before being advised by a medical expert. So, while it is safe to practice intermittent fasting and include exercise if you are an already active person, doing so is not suitable for everyone.

First of all, your metabolism can be negatively impacted if you exercise and fast for long periods. For example, if you exercise daily while fasting for more than a month, your metabolic rate can begin to slow down. So while it may sound like a quick way to reap the benefits of your limited calorie intake, moderation is crucial.

Combining the two can trigger a higher rate of breaking down glycogen and body fat. This means that you burn fat at an accelerated rate. Also, when you combine these two, your growth hormones are boosted. This results in improved bone density. Your muscles are also positively impacted when you exercise. Your muscles will become more resilient to stress and age slower. This is also a quick way to trigger autophagy keeping brain cells and tissues strong, making you feel, and look younger.

Exercise is Even Better After 50

Cardiovascular exercise is great for the heart and lungs. It improves oxygen delivery to specific parts of your body, reduces stress, improves sleep, burns fat, and improves sex drive. Some of the more common cardio exercises are running, brisk walking, and swimming. In the gym, machines such as the elliptical, treadmill, and stairmaster are used to help with cardio. Some people are satisfied and feel like they've done enough after 20 minutes on the treadmill, but if you want to continue to be strong and independent as you grow older, you need to consider adding strength training to your workout. After 50, strength training for a woman is no longer about six-pack abs, building biceps, or vanity muscles. Instead, it has switched to maintaining a body that is healthy, strong, and is less prone to injury and illness.

Women over 50 who engage in strength training for 20 to 30 minutes a day can reap the following benefits:

1. **Reduced body fat**: Accumulating excess body fat is not healthy for any woman at any age. To prevent many of the diseases associated with aging, it is important to maintain a healthy body weight by burning excess fat.

2. **Build bone density**: With stronger bones, accidental falls are less likely to result in broken limbs or a visit to the emergency room..

3. **Build muscle mass**: Although you are not likely to be the next champion bodybuilder, strength training will make you an overall stronger woman who will carry herself with ease, push your lawnmower, lift your groceries, and perform all other tasks that require you to exert some strength.

4. **Significant less risk of chronic diseases**: In addition to keeping chronic diseases away, strength training can also reduce symptoms of some diseases you may have, such as back pain, obesity, arthritis, osteoporosis, and diabetes. Of course, the type of exercises you do if you have any chronic disease should be recommended by your doctor.

5. **Boosts mental health**: A loss of self-confidence and depression are some psychological issues that come along with aging. Women who keep themselves fit with exercises tend to be generally more self-assured and are less likely to develop depression.

Strength Training Exercises for Women Over 50

These ten strength training exercises you can do right in the comfort of your home. All you need is a mat, a chair, and some hand weights of about 3 – 8 pounds. As you get stronger, you can increase the weight. Take a minute to rest before switching between each routine. Ensure that you move slowly through the exercises, breathe properly, and focus on maintaining the right form. If you start to feel lightheaded or dizzy during your routines, especially if you are performing the exercise during your fasting window, discontinue immediately.

<u>Squat to Chair</u>

This exercise is great for improving your bone health. A lot of age-related bone fractures and falls in women involve the pelvis, so this exercise will target and strengthen your pelvic bone and the surrounding muscles.

To perform this:

1. Stand fully upright in front of a chair as if you are ready to sit and spread your feet shoulder-width apart.
2. Extend your arms in front of you and keep them that way all through the movement.
3. Bend your knees and slowly lower your hips as if you want to sit on the chair, but don't sit. When your butt touches the chair slightly, press into your heels to get back your initial standing position. Repeat that for about 10 to 15 times.

Forearm Plank

This exercise targets your core and shoulders.

Here's how to do it:

1. Get into a push-up position, but with your arms bent at the elbows such that your forearm is supporting your weight.
2. Keep your body off the mat or floor and keep your back straight at all times. Don't raise or drop your hips. This will engage your core. Hold the position for 30 seconds and then drop to your knees. Repeat ten times.

Modified Push-ups

This routine targets your arms, shoulders, and core.

How's how to do it:

1. Kneel on your mat. Place your hands on the mat below your shoulders and let your knees be behind your hips so that your back is stretched at an angle.
2. Tuck your toes under and tighten your abdominal muscles. Gradually bend your elbows as you lower your chest toward the floor.
3. Push back on your arms to press your chest back to your previous position. Repeat for as many times as is comfortable.

Bird Dog

When done correctly, this exercise can strengthen the muscles of your posterior chain as it targets your back and core. It may seem easy at first but can be a bit tricky.

To do this correctly:

1. Go on all fours on your mat.
2. Tighten your abdominal muscles and shift your weight to your right knee and left hand. Slowly extend your right hand in front of

you and your left leg behind you. Ensure that both your hands and legs are extended as far as possible and stay in that position for about 5 seconds. Return to your starting position. This is one repetition. Switch to your left knee and right hand and repeat the movement. Alternate between both sides for 20 repetitions.

Shoulder Overhead Press

This targets your biceps, shoulders, and back.

To perform this move:

1. With dumbbells in both hands, stand and spread your feet shoulder-width apart.
2. Bring the dumbbells up to the sides of your head and tighten your abdominal muscles.
3. Slowly press the dumbbells up until your arms are straight above your head. Slowly return to the first position. Repeat 10 times. You can also do this exercise while sitting.

Chest Fly

This targets your chest, back, core, and glutes.

To do this:

1. Lie with your back flat on your mat, your knees at an angle close to 90 degrees, and your feet firmly planted on the floor or mat.
2. Hold dumbbells in both hands over your chest. Keep your palms facing each other and gently open your hands away from your chest. Let your upper arms touch the floor without releasing the tension in them.
3. Contract your chest muscles and slowly return the dumbbells to the initial position. Repeat for about ten times.

Standing Calf Raise

This exercise improves the mobility of your lower legs and feet and also improves your stability.

Here's how to perform it.

- Hold a dumbbell in your left hand and place your right hand on something sturdy to give you balance.
- When you are sure of your balance, lift your left foot off the floor with the dumbbell hanging at your side. Stand erect and move

your weight such that you are almost standing on your toes.

- Slowly return to the starting position. Do this 15 times before switching to the other leg and doing the same thing all over again.

Single-Leg Hamstring Bridge

This move targets your glutes, quads, and hamstrings.

To do this:

1. Lie flat on your back. Place your feet flat on the floor or mat and spread your bent knees apart.
2. Place your arms flat by your side and lift one leg straight.
3. Contract your glutes as you lift your hips into a bridge position with your arms still in position. Hold for about 2 to 3 seconds and drop your hips to the mat. Repeat about ten times before switching your leg. Do the same again.

Bent-Over Row

This targets your back muscles and spine.

To do this:

1. Hold dumbbells in both hands and stand behind a sturdy object (for example, a chair). Bend forward and rest your head on the chosen object. Relax your neck and slightly bend your knees. With both palms facing each other pull the dumbbells to touch your ribs. Hold the position for about 2 to 5 seconds and slowly return to the starting position. Repeat 10 to 15 times.

Basic Ab

A distended belly is a common occurrence in older women. This exercise can strengthen and tighten the abdominal muscles bringing them inward toward your spine.

To perform this:

1. Lie on your back with your feet firmly planted on the floor and your knees bent. Relax your upper body and rest your hands on your thighs.
2. As you exhale, lift yourself upward off the mat or floor. Stop the upward movement

when your hands are resting on your knees. Hold the position for about 2 to 5 seconds and then slowly return to the starting position. Repeat for about 20 to 30 times.

Include Exercises in Your Daily Routine

You do not have to hit the gym or plan a time dedicated to working out. You can make exercise part of your daily routine so that you are always getting the proper amount of body movement, whether or not it is time for exercise.

Here are a few tips on how to include exercises into your daily routine.

- Take the stairs (within reason) instead of using the elevator. You don't want to go up a ten-story building using the stairs! If you have a long way to go up or down, take the stairs a couple of flights and then complete your trip with the elevator.
- When you talk with your family members at home, don't shout from the top floor and bottom floor. Go up or climb down and talk with them.
- Find a sporting activity that you thoroughly enjoy and do it as often as is convenient. When you're doing something you enjoy,

you'll hardly think of it as exercise, and you're likely to stay committed.

- If you are at work, instead of sending emails or text messages to coworkers, walk up to them and talk to them face to face.
- If possible, convert your one-on-one meetings to a walking meeting. Hold the meeting while taking a stroll outside.
- Stop a block or two from your destination and walk the rest of the way. Make walking your preferred mode of transportation.
- Take your dog for walks daily. If you don't have a dog, adopt one. It might seem that you are merely walking your dog, but you are exercising your muscles.
- Take brisk walks as often as possible. Remember to put on comfortable shoes when walking briskly. You can bring your walking shoes with you to make it easy for you to change into them.

Staying Safe While Combining Intermittent Fasting and Exercise

Exercising in your fasting window can help you quickly achieve some of the advanced benefits of intermittent fasting. Nevertheless, it is crucial to follow a few general guidelines to keep you safe during the practice.

There are no iron-cast rules about when to exercise even on fasting days. Observe what works well for you – whether exercising before eating (during the fasting window) or eating before working out (during the eating window). Many women find that exercising on an empty stomach suits their body and leaves them feeling energized for the rest of the day. If this is your, set aside time in the morning before your first meal of the day. Some other women find that although they prefer working out on an empty stomach, they feel depleted right after the exercise. In that case, shift your exercise to about 20 to 30 minutes before your first meal of the day. Your body would have rested a bit after your exercise before you break your fast.

If you prefer working out after you break your fast, that is perfectly fine. Eating shortly before your exercise doesn't render your exercises ineffective. Remember that all of our bodies work in different ways. Keep in mind that the goal of working out is to maintain proper body health long into your golden years. You don't need to impress anyone with great abs or biceps, instead impress yourself with how much power you have. Stay committed to your routines, but don't over do it. If you start feeling weak, that is your cue to take a break.

If you are fasting for longer periods (24 hours or more), you will need to conserve your energy.

Consider doing exercises that will not exert too much stress. Take a walk, do some yoga, or any other type of low-intensity exercise.

We could all use someone on our shoulder reminding us to drink more water. And going without food reduces your body's water content even more. Add in higher levels of exertion and you'll be depleting your water reserves very quickly. So here is your reminder to always drink adequate amounts of water before, during, and after your workout sessions.

Chapter 5:

Activating Autophagy

What if there is a way to stay forever young? What if you could erase a couple of years from your face and skin and take off some inches from your waistline by activating an internal cleanup process? Would you not want to know how to do that? Well, staying forever young or finding a literal fountain of youth might be unlikely but you can stimulate a natural process to keep cells rejuvenated and functioning optimally for the rest of your life. That process is known as autophagy.

What is Autophagy and How Does It Work?

Reduce, reuse, and recycle is a popular phrase you're likely to hear in discussions relating to environmental sustainability. This is similar in many ways to what autophagy does – reducing or breaking down and repairing parts of your cells, and then recycling important body chemicals that can be reused by the liver.

In a nutshell, autophagy is the natural process that removes toxic materials and broken cells from your body to create new and healthier cells. The term comes from Latin which translates to self-eating (*auto*="self" and *phagy*="to eat"). In a weird way, this means your body is eating itself! Don't panic, it's a good thing. It's a rejuvenation process for your body.

If you fully realize what autophagy is and how to make it work for you, you will be quick to find ways to consciously stimulate the process because it can keep you feeling and looking younger than your real age! Older adults, in particular, can use this natural process to increase longevity.

Here's a simple analogy of how autophagy works that I think a lot of women can relate to. Think of what happens inside your kitchen when you are preparing a delicious meal. You are creating something heartfelt and necessary while at the same time making a mess and producing waste. If you leave your kitchen dirty after preparing your meal, it will be difficult to make your next meal. So you do what any self-respecting woman does: throw or put away leftovers, clean the counter, put away unused ingredients, and recycle some of the food if you can. This is exactly how autophagy works in your body. It cleans up after you!

A big mess is created each day inside the body. This mess includes parts of dead cells, damaged proteins, and harmful particles that prevent optimal body function. When you were much younger, the process of autophagy clears this mess up as quickly as possible, keeping them looking young and supple. But as you grow older, the cleanup process slows down. Dirt, mess, and crumbs start to build up internally due to old age. If left unattended, the buildup can result in rapid aging, increased risk of cancer and dementia, as well as other diseases associated with old age.

But growing older doesn't mean you're doomed to have an inefficient cellular cleaning process. You can stimulate the process of autophagy and make it work as it used to when you were a lot younger. An effective way to do that is by doing something that induces stress such as decreasing insulin levels and increasing your glucagon levels. In simpler terms, go without food for longer than you usually would. When you get really hungry as you do when you fast, your glucagon is increased and stimulates autophagy.

You can achieve some positive life-altering benefits by simply activating autophagy. But before going into the immense health benefits, let us consider the science behind the process, albeit briefly.

The Science Behind Autophagy

Autophagy in humans is induced by the activation of a protein known as p62. As soon as broken or damaged cells caused by metabolic byproducts begin to appear, p62 stimulates the process of clearing up the clutter on a cellular level. All remaining parts of waste, or damaged cells that can lead to health problems are reduced, reused, and recycled. Think of the process as decluttering on a cellular level. The entire process is neatly executed to keep you healthy, strong to handle any biological stress, and of course, keep you looking and feeling young.

Researchers from Newcastle University found that humans evolved to live longer by responding well to biological stressors (Newcastle University, 2018). Usually, fruit flies can't withstand stress. But when researchers genetically altered fruit flies by giving them the human version of p62, they found that the fruit flies lived longer than usual even under stressful conditions. The lead author in the study, Dr. Vicktor Korolchuk, aptly concluded, *"This tells us that abilities, like sensing stress and activating protective processes like autophagy, may have evolved to allow better stress resistance and a longer lifespan."*

The Benefits

Some people are said to have different biological and chronological age. That is to say, their age is different from their quality of their life. Women are more likely to worry about showing signs of aging or looking older than men. Thankfully, you can look younger by activating autophagy. What the process does to your cells is to remove toxins and recycle cells instead of creating new ones. These rejuvenated cells will behave like new and work better.

Your skin is constantly exposed to harmful lights, air, chemicals, as well as harsh weather conditions. This causes damage to your skin cells. As the damaged cells continue to accumulate, your skin begins to wrinkle, lose elasticity, and no longer appear smooth. The process of autophagy repairs your skin cells that might have been partly damaged to make your skin glow and healthier. In the same way that wear and tear happens with things you use frequently, wear and tear (microtear) also happens to your muscles as you use them especially during exercises. Your muscles become inflamed and require repairs. What this means is you need more energy to use these specific muscles. The process of autophagy in your cells will degrade the damaged parts in the muscle, reduce the amount of energy sent to the muscle, and ensure energy balance.

To keep your metabolism working well, your cells need to be in top shape. The powerhouse of your cell is the mitochondria. A lot of harmful trash is left behind in the mitochondria as it performs its function of burning fat and making adenosine triphosphate (ATP) – the molecule that stores all the energy you need to do almost everything. This harmful trash can damage your cells. Autophagy ensures that these toxins are promptly taken care of to prevent damage to your cells and keep them in a healthy state.

Several processes and activities that occur during your cellular cleaning and repairs also help you to maintain a healthy weight. For example, when toxins are removed from your cells through autophagy and you successfully excrete them, your fat cells can no longer store these toxins. Also, when you fast for short periods (12 to 16 hours), autophagy is activated, fat-burning also takes place, and since it is not a prolonged fast, your proteins are spared. All these activities and processes help to make you leaner and fitter.

The cells of your gastrointestinal tract hardly ever take breaks. You put them to work consistently, and this can affect digestive health. Autophagy helps repair and restore the cells. When you stop eating for long periods you give your gut ample time to rest and heal. Giving your gut some rest (from digesting your meal) is vital for an overall improved digestive health.

Certain neurodegenerative diseases such as Alzheimer's disease and Parkinson's disease are a result of too much accumulation of damaged proteins around the brain cells. Autophagy clears this clutter of damaged proteins that don't work as they should. Dementia is not a normal part of aging, even though it is largely linked to older people. You can keep all these diseases at bay by activating autophagy. If your brain cells are clear of clutter (damaged protein cells), you will perform cognitive functions optimally.

How to Activate Autophagy

As already stated, one of the quickest ways to activate autophagy is by staying away from food for longer periods. In other words, intermittent fasting can create just the right level of stress on your body to kick start the internal cleanup process. Going without food leads to an energy deficit, and that induces autophagy ridding your body of decaying cells and accumulated junk. So, besides the widely known weight loss benefits of intermittent fasting, perhaps a far-reaching positive aspect of practicing intermittent fasting is activating autophagy.

Physical exercise is another stress-inducing activity that can stimulate autophagy. This is particularly true for areas of the body where the process of metabolic regulation occurs. Some of these areas of the body where exercise-induced autophagy is the liver, muscles, and pancreas.

When you combine intermittent fasting with moderate physical exercises (as suggested in the previous chapter), you are taking autophagy to a new level. And considering all the benefits that you get from autophagy, isn't it worth giving up snacking after dinner?

Chapter 6:
Practical Tips for Fasting

Practice indeed makes perfect. To help you get in the intermittent fasting, I have outlined a few down-to-earth routes and hands-on tips to guide you. Your approach to fasting can mean the difference between success and failure. So, consider these tips as guidelines that will help safely implement your preferred fasting regimen.

Find a Worthy Goal

First things first: find a goal that is worth pursuing, or else you will drop the idea at the first sign of resistance. If you don't have a goal that represents a strong ideal, it won't be long before you start telling yourself, "*I think I've passed the stage of such childishness.*" And yes, many women start a new lifestyle change for reasons that they can't keep up when things get tough. For example, the desire to look like models on TV, or social media makes losing weight feel socially acceptable, and ok to keep up with trends that can be harmful. These reasons are not enough to keep anyone committed to a full lifestyle change and few wonder why so many people with goals are quick to jump from one lifestyle to another.

Don't go into fasting intermittently because it is the thing to do at the moment. Instead, look for inspiring goals such as:

- Staying fit, young, and healthy.
- Improving your cognitive or brain functions.
- Improving your overall vitality and increase energy levels.
- Balancing hormones, especially during menopausal or post-menopausal stages of life.
- Improving your overall health, thereby increasing longevity.

Do any of these sound good to you? Surely at this stage of your life, you are aware of the inherent risks of doing something merely because others are doing it too. That type of motivation will fail you.

Check Your Hormones

A woman's hormones can be easily thrown out of whack by the slightest change in her already established pattern of behavior. Whether it is a physical change such as altering your eating pattern or an emotional change such as being irritated or sad, it can bring about hormonal imbalance in a woman even if it is temporary.

But for the perimenopausal and menopausal women, hormones can go haywire for reasons even they can't define. She could be feeling really great all week, and without anything changing she could suddenly become fatigued, depressed, and not in the right frame of mind. These changes happen due to the unpredictability of this phase of a woman's life. Because this can happen for no apparent reason, it is best to check your hormonal levels before putting your body through a major lifestyle change. If you've ever had issues with thyroid, cortisol, or adrenal fatigue, ensure that you have these checks before you begin.

This may come as a surprise to some women, but your ovaries produce testosterone too. So, as you grow older and begin to experience a decline in your estrogen and progesterone levels, your testosterone levels are also taking a nosedive. Your libido can be affected by low levels of testosterone and make you feel exhausted and bummed-out for no reason at all. So while you are checking your other hormones, don't forget to do a testosterone test. The thyroid and testosterone hormones also help in weight regulation. So, if you intend to shed some weight using intermittent fasting, these tests are very necessary.

Start Slow

To go from having five or six meals daily to eating only once a day can lead to very dire consequences. In addition to being harmful to your health, massive abrupt changes are hardly sustainable. After confirming that intermittent fasting is suitable for your health, the next thing to do is planning how to ease into the habit. Take another look at the example of how to ease into fasting in Chapter 2 and consider following the example or coming up with something similar that works for you. In other words, before you fully implement any intermittent fasting regimen, it is a good practice to first test the waters, so to speak, with a less strict form of fasting. By doing this, it will help your body acclimate to the changes before going into the proper regimen.

Don't Fuss Over What You Can Eat

One common mistake people make when fasting is obsessing over the fasting hours and what to eat when they are finally allowed. You don't have to worry about if you are fasting as long as someone else, the important thing is what's comfortable for you. Of course, if your fasting window is too small, you are not likely to see any result. Also, don't get too tied up in every little detail of intermittent fasting. For example, you don't have to become too worried because you missed a day. Remember that fasting intermittently should be a lifestyle change if you want to continue to reap the benefits. And for a lifestyle change to be sustainable, you must be able to adapt and use it in a way that even if you face challenges, you will work your way around it somehow. Missing a day or cutting your fast short for reasons beyond your control shouldn't get you worked up and worrying about whether you can do the entire plan. Don't give up.

Again, some people focus too much on what they can eat or not eat. For example, *"Can I add just a little butter or cream?"* *"Would it hurt to eat this type of food during the fasting window?"* If your focus is on what you can have or eat while you are fasting, you are giving your attention to the wrong things and putting your mind in an unhelpful state. Give your mind the right focus by concentrating on doing a good, clean, fast, and try to consume only water, tea, or coffee during the window.

Watch Electrolytes

Your body electrolytes are compounds and elements that occur naturally in body fluids, blood, and urine. They can also be ingested through drinks, foods, and supplements. Some of them include magnesium, calcium, potassium, chloride, phosphate, and sodium. Their functions include fluid balance, regulation of the heart and neurological function, acid-base balance, oxygen delivery, and many other functions.

It is important to keep these electrolytes in a state of balance. But many people who practice fasting tend to neglect this and run into problems. Here is a common notion: "Don't let anything into your stomach until the end of your fast" Even those just starting to fast know it doesn't work that way, and they tend to forget or fully stay away from liquids during their fasting window.

When you lose too much water from your body through sweating, vomiting, and diarrhea, or you don't have enough water in your body because you don't drink enough liquids, you increase the risk of electrolyte disorders. It is not okay to drink tea or black coffee throughout the morning period of your fast window. You will wear yourself down if you don't drink enough water. The longer you fast without water, the higher your chances of flushing out electrolytes and running into trouble. You can end up raising your blood pressure, develop muscle twitching and spasms, fatigue, fast heart rate or irregular heartbeat, and many other health problems.

On the other hand, drinking too much water can also tip the water-electrolyte balance. What you want to do is to drink adequate amounts of water

and not excess water, whether you are fasting or
not.

Give the Calorie Restriction a Rest

Remember that intermittent fasting is different
from dieting. Your focus should be on eating
healthily during your eating window or eating days
instead of focusing on calorie restriction. Even if
you are fasting for weight loss, don't obsess over
calories. Following a fasting regimen is enough to
take care of the calories you consume. It is
absolutely unnecessary to engage in a practice that
can hurt your metabolism. Combining intermittent
fasting with eating too little food in your eating
window because you are worried about your calorie
intake can cause problems for your metabolism.

One of the major reasons that people push
themselves into restricting calories while fasting is
their concern for rapid weight loss. You need to be
wary of any process that brings about drastic
physical changes to your body in very short
amounts of time. While it is okay to desire quick
results, your health and safety are more important.
When you obsess or worry that you are not losing
weight as quickly as you want, you are not helping
matters. Instead, you are increasing your stress
level, and that is counterproductive. You are already
taking practical steps toward losing weight by

intermittent fasting, why would you want to undo your hard work by unnecessary worrying?

Simply focus on following a sustainable intermittent fasting regimen and let go of the need to restrict your calorie intake. Intermittent fasting will give your body the right number of calories it needs if you do it properly.

The First Meal of the Eating Window Is Key

Breaking your fast is a crucial part of the process because if you don't get it right, it could quickly develop into unhealthy eating patterns. When you break your fast, it is important to have healthy foods around to prevent grabbing unhealthy feel good snacks. Make sure what you are eating in your window is not a high-sugar or high-carb meal. I recommend that you consider breaking your fast with something that is highly nutrient-dense such as a green smoothie, protein shake, or healthy salad.

As much as possible, avoid breaking your fast with foods from a fast-food restaurant. Eating junk foods after your fast is a quick way to ruin all the hard work you've put in during your fasting window. If, for any reason, you can't prepare your meal, ensure that you order very specific foods that will complement your effort and not destroy what you've built.

Break Your Fast Gently

It is okay to feel very hungry after going for a long time without food, even if you were drinking water all through the fasting window. This is particularly true for people who are just starting with fasting. But don't let the intensity of your hunger push you to eat. You don't want to force food hurriedly into your stomach after going long without food, or you might hurt yourself and experience stomach distress. Take it slow when you break your fast. Eat light meals in small portions first when you break your fast. Wait for a couple of minutes for your stomach to get used to the presence of food again before continuing with a normal-sized meal. The waiting period will douse any hunger pangs and remove the urge to rush your meal. For example, break your fast with a small serving of salad and wait for about 15 minutes. Drink some water and then after about five more minutes, you can eat a normal-sized meal.

Nutrition is Important

Although intermittent fasting is not dieting and so, does not specify which foods to eat, limit, and completely avoid, it makes sense to eat healthily. This means focusing on eating a balanced diet, such as:

1. Whole grains
2. Fruits and vegetables (canned in water, fresh, or frozen).
3. Lean sources of protein (lentils, beans, eggs, poultry, tofu, and so on).
4. Healthy fats (nuts, seeds, coconuts, avocados, olive oil, olive, and fatty fish).

It simply doesn't make any sense to go for 16 hours (or more) without food and then spend the rest of the day eating junk. Even if you follow the 5:2 diet and limit your calorie intake to only 500 calories per day for two days, it is totally illogical to follow it with five days of eating highly processed foods and low-quality meals. Combining intermittent fasting with unbalanced diets will lead to nutritional deficiencies and defeat the goal of fasting in the first place. Realize that intermittent fasting is not a magic wand that makes all poor eating habits vanish in a poof! For the practice to work, you must be deliberate about the types of food you eat.

Find a Regimen That Works for You

Don't follow a fasting diet because it seems to suit someone else. Instead, go for something that fits into your schedule. If you feel caged or boxed in by a particular fasting plan, it is a clear indication that it is not a suitable plan for you. Thankfully, you have the freedom to design something that works for you, even if you are following a specific regimen. The regimens are not carved in stone! They are flexible, and you can adjust them to suit you as long as you follow each regimen's basic principles. For example, if you decide to follow the 16:8 fasting regimen, your 8-hour eating window must not strictly be between noon and 8 pm. You have the option of tailoring the eating window to something that gives you room to handle other aspects of your life, such as work, hobbies, family, and so on. You might decide to make your 8-hour eating window from 9 am to 5 pm, or from 1 pm to 9 pm.

Whatever you choose to do is totally up to you. After all, it is your life, and you have the freedom to choose what you want. Books, the internet, and even loved ones can only suggest and offer recommendations. Ultimately, the final decision rests with you. Since your goal is not to please someone else or seek external approval, you should make your choice based on what is most convenient for you. You are seeking results, not accolades.

Therefore, don't follow something unrealistic for you or too restrictive. Even if you endure the most stringent type of fast and get admiration and commendation from others, have you considered what that fasting regimen is doing to your overall health? The female body is delicately designed, and putting it through unnecessary stress is unsafe if you are merely enduring discomfort to boost your ego.

Be Patient

Whatever propaganda you may have heard about fast results, the reality is that nothing is typical because we all have unique processes regardless of our physical appearance. Be patient even if others who began fasting at the same time are already seeing results and you have nothing to show for your efforts so far. It can be frustrating and discouraging but give your body time to adjust. As long as you don't have any medical reason to stop, don't give up just yet. Continue the practice for at least a month.

Realize that changes take time. There is no magic about the process of losing weight, improved vitality, or any other health benefits of intermittent fasting. Don't be in a hurry, and don't give people the room to put you under unnecessary pressure. Each person has their own pace, and it has absolutely nothing to do with you. If you continue to focus on other people's results or your seeming lack of results, you are giving your mind reasons to discontinue. Be patient.

What To Eat

I have reiterated the need to eat healthily during your eating window. This section will give you some great ideas on the types of food you can eat to help you achieve your health goals faster and maintain an overall healthy body. Several healthy foods too numerous to list here are excellent for intermittent fasting. In addition to these, consider including the following to your shopping list:

- Fish contains good amounts of vitamin D and is rich in proteins and fat. Fish is good for your brain, and since lower calorie intake due to fasting can disrupt your cognition, fish is a great addition to your food cart.
- Cauliflower, Brussels sprouts, broccoli, and other cruciferous veggies. Besides making you feel full (which is how you definitely want to feel if you are going to stay away from eating for 16 long hours!), they can help to prevent constipation during fasting because they are rich in fiber.

- Beans and legumes are low in carbs and can keep your energy up during fasting. Black beans, peas, chickpeas, and lentils can also help in reducing your body weight even when you are not restricting your calorie intake.
- Avocado contains high calories, but the monounsaturated fat in it can keep you full for a long time.
- Whole grains may sound out of place when trying to lose weight because they contain carbs. But they are also rich in protein and fiber. When you eat whole grains instead of refined grains, you are helping to improve your metabolism. So go for whole grains such as millet, brown rice, oatmeal, spelt, farro, amaranth, whole-wheat bread, and bulgur. As much as possible, limit refined grains such as white flour, white bread, white rice, and degermed cornflower.
- Probiotic-rich foods such as kombucha, kefir, tempeh, and miso are excellent for your gut health.

Chapter 7:
Dealing with Unpleasant Side Effects

Earlier in the introduction, I promised you unbiased information on intermittent fasting. In keeping with that promise, this chapter will delve into the possible negative side effects of fasting intermittently. Some people who swear by this practice may not be willing to admit that there are unpleasant side effects of fasting intermittently. But that would be myopic and withholding vital information.

Having said that, it is important to point out that the general downsides of intermittent fasting are common to all women regardless of age. While women of child-bearing age might have effects on their reproductive hormones, post-menopausal women or older women may not need to worry about reproduction, although they experience frequent changes in their moods, difficulty in sleeping, and occasional headaches.

After a comprehensive review of several scientific studies on women's health, fasting, and aging, researchers weren't able to find any significant negative effect of intermittent fasting and point to a lack of research on the topic (Journal of Mid-Life Health, 2016). These types of scientific reviews are very useful for getting the unbiased information that gives you a broader picture of several results from different related studies performed over many years. Comprehensive reviews cut down prejudices often associated with smaller studies that may have been sponsored by special interest groups. Overall, scientific studies show encouraging results in different aspects of women's health including mental health, physical health, and weight loss. That is not to say, there are no negative side effects of intermittent fasting. It only means that the negative side effects of intermittent fasting are common to women of all ages – both pre and post-menopausal women and depend largely on the individual woman.

With that being said, not everyone who practices intermittent fasting will have a negative side effect. These differ from person to person. The important thing is being aware of these negative side effects and learning how to handle them if they occur. Also, remember that most of the off-putting effects of intermittent fast don't last beyond the first few days. Within a week or two, your body would have adjusted to your new eating schedule and any negative effects will gradually subside until things feel back to normal. So it is important to allow your body some time to adjust instead of trying intermittent fasting for one or two days and throwing in the towel.

Here is how to deal with some of the common negative side effects you will likely encounter as you start your new eating habits.

Hunger

One of the first not-so-fun and most obvious results of fasting is hunger. This side effect is difficult because going without food longer than your body is conditioned to will result in an uncomfortable desire for anything to eat. All your life, you have programmed your body to expect food at certain times throughout the day. It would be weird if you suddenly change your eating pattern, and your body accepts the change without putting up at least a little resistance. If your body doesn't get food at the time it normally does, a hormone called ghrelin – the hunger hormone – will start acting up to remind you that you should supply your body with food. This "acting up" or reminder to eat at your usual time will continue until your brain convinces ghrelin to accept your new eating schedule. But until then, you will likely feel intense hunger but don't worry it will pass. You will need to tap into your reserve of mental strength to stay committed to your course.

To effectively handle hunger pangs, drink more water, or any qualifying beverage on intermittent fasting. Doing so will help to suppress hunger pangs. Quite often, the feeling of hunger is not necessarily an indication that you are hungry; it might be a slight dip in your blood sugar level – something that water or other non-calorie liquids can take care of.

To help delay hunger on your fasting days or during the fasting window (depending on the type of fasting regimen you choose to follow), ensure that you include adequate amounts of healthy fats, carbs, and proteins in your meals before commencing your fast. Also, during your fast, try to keep your mind off food. Combining low-impact exercises with fasting can help give you the boost you need to go through your day without feeling too uncomfortable. Getting enough sleep will also help you throughout the day; there is nothing that will upset your day more than lack of sleep at night and having to fast. That is an open invitation for fatigue and hunger!

Frequent Urination

As with hunger, it is also expected to experience an increase in the number of times you urinate. There is no mystery here as intermittent fasting requires that you increase your intake of water and other liquids to stay hydrated. This will in turn increase the frequency of urination. Keep drinking your water and don't avoid bathroom visits. Holding it for too long can weaken your bladder muscles and trying not to drink water will soon make you dehydrated and provide the next side effect – both bad!

Headaches

Intermittent fasting can make your blood sugar to take a nosedive. This introduces stress on your body, your brain will release stress hormones, and you will likely experience some degree of headache. Dehydration can lead to headaches during intermittent fasting as your body it is telling you it lacks adequate water.

To reduce the occurrence of headaches, try to minimize stress on your body. It is okay to exercise during fasting, but excessive exercise can trigger a large amount of stress. Also, try to keep your body hydrated at all times by drinking enough water. But don't chug water in a rush and don't drink water excessively. Too much water can result in an imbalance in your mineral and body water ratio.

Cravings

It is normal to experience more than usual cravings for food during your fasting window. This is a biological and psychological response to the feeling of deprivation that is often associated with going without food. And because your body is all out to get glucose, you might notice that you crave for more sugar or carbohydrates. These cravings don't mean that you are less committed to your goals. Rather, cravings happen to remind you that you are human. Even ardent practitioners of intermittent fasting experience cravings from time to time.

When you start craving for something, remind yourself of your goal and distract yourself from food-related topics. Keep your mind engrossed with other non-food related activities such as hobbies, talking a walk in nature, or going to sleep for a while. During your eating window, you can treat yourself to a healthy bite of what you crave to minimize the intensity of the craving or longing. Remind yourself during your fasting window that you will soon eat what you long for, so there's no need dwelling on it or giving it too much thought when it is not yet time to eat. Remind your body that you are no longer a teenager or a young adult. You have had lots of experience in curbing your cravings, and this case is not an exception.

Heartburn, Bloating, and Constipation

Occasionally, heartburn can occur when your stomach produces acids for digestion of your food, but there is no food present in the stomach to be digested. Bloating and constipation usually go hand in hand and can also occur in some cases. Together, these two can make you feel very uncomfortable.

Drinking adequate amounts of water can reduce the risk of heartburn, bloating, and constipation. Heartburns can also be minimized by cutting down on spicy foods during your eating window. If you experience heartburn during intermittent fasting, here's something you can try before going to sleep. Prop yourself up when you lie down to sleep. But don't use pillows to prop yourself as that will put more pressure on your stomach and increase the discomfort. Use a specially designed wedge or use a 6-inch block or something similar to elevate your head as you lie down. Doing this will make gravity minimize the backward flow of your stomach contents into your gullet. Propping yourself this way should bring you relief from heartburn. However, if heartburn, bloating, and constipation persist, consult your doctor immediately.

Binging

Eating a large amount as soon as the fasting window is over is usually associated with first-timers to fasting. The intense hunger of fasting can drive you to eat in a hurry when breaking, and you can end up overeating. In some cases, binging can be a result of a simple misunderstanding of the basics of intermittent fasting. They assume that they can eat as much as they want in the eating window since the no-eating window will take care of calories. This misunderstanding can deprive you of gaining any significant benefits that come with fasting intermittently, especially if you are looking to shed some weight. Binging or overeating in your eating window will reverse all the hard work you put in during the fast.

To avoid binging, ensure that the size and type of meal is planned well ahead of the eating window. Don't start fasting without knowing what portion you are going to consume at the end. Waiting until you can eat to decide what to eat and how much to eat can lead to overeating because your food choices will be largely influenced by how hungry you feel.

Low Energy

Feeling exhausted is a normal part of fasting. Until your body gets used to sourcing its fuel from fat storage, you are likely to experience some decline in your energy levels. Usually, they get back up within a couple of days.

To help stay energized, tailor your activities to remain low-key, at least at first. There is no need to push yourself to prove that you are a strong woman. Deciding to practice intermittent fasting is enough proof that you are mentally, emotionally, and physically strong. Since you are not in competition with anyone, it is in your best interest to conserve energy as much as possible. Get a massage, spend time relaxing in bed, or sleeping in if you have to. These little activities can go a long way in keeping you energized.

Feeling Cold

Some people experience an extra feeling of cold during fasting. If you experience this, there is no cause for alarm. It might be a result of the drop in your blood sugar level. Usually, blood flow to your internal fat storage is increased during fasting. As a result of this increase, your fat is moved to parts of your body where it needs to be used as energy. This can make other parts of your body that have less fat storage to experience cold. So if you feel cold in your fingers or toes, it is your body doing its fat burning process for your own good.

To help reduce the cold, put on layers, stay in warm places, drink hot coffee or tea (with no calories), or take a hot shower. It is important to keep in mind that feeling cold is just a result of intermittent fasting and does not mean you are ill. So avoid the urge to self-medicate. If the cold feeling persists even in your non-fasting days or in your eating window, consult your doctor.

Mood Swing

Imagine the following combinations. Stress on your body caused by the dip in your blood sugar. Your hormones are going berserk from the various reactions going on in your body as a result of not eating normally, or on schedule. The lethargic feeling from lack of food, hunger, and cravings constantly telling you to eat. Not being able to socialize with others freely because of your new eating pattern you can't wine and dine at social events if it is outside your eating window! All of these can lead to a psychological state of feeling annoyed or irritated.

The surest way to minimize mood swings resulting from intermittent fasting is to deliberately keep your attention off issues that set you on edge and focus on what you are doing and what makes you happy. The more you keep your mind wrapped up in gratitude and appreciation, the better you will feel. So, during your fasting window, be deliberate about engaging in things that lift your spirits and keep your mind on happy and productive thoughts.

Bottom Line

Intermittent fasting is a lifestyle regimen that is safe for older practitioners. It is a medical intervention that can bring about improvements in many aspects of a woman's health. However, it is not suitable for every person. If you notice that you have severe negative reactions to intermittent fasting, it is in your best interest to desist at once and consult your doctor. No rule makes it compulsory to complete a fast once you begin. You can absolutely break in the middle of your fasting window (even if it is just that day) if you can no longer endure an unpleasant side effects and try again at a later time.

While it is okay to give your body a few weeks to get used to your new eating pattern, it is also crucial to pay close attention to what your body is telling you. Thankfully, as an older woman with experience, you can tell when something works for you or not. You know when you can commit to something and when you can't find the motivation to follow through. I believe that, as a woman with a tremendous wealth of experience, you will find the strength to stick to your resolve within reason.

Chapter 8:
Busting the Myths

Issues that are not popular can be misunderstood with a lot of misconceptions and myths surrounding them. Intermittent fasting is one such issue. Many people with half-baked information suddenly become experts on the topic and are always willing to give advice to anyone willing to listen. This chapter debunks some of these myths. It doesn't matter how long a false premise is considered correct, once the evidence is present, the error is exposed and wise people will know to stick with the facts.

Myth #1: Intermittent Fasting Is Unsafe for Older Adults

Anyone can engage in intermittent fasting as long as they do not have any medical conditions and are not pregnant or lactating. Of course, our bodies do not all have the same tolerance levels even in people that look exactly alike. If one or more persons respond negatively to intermittent fasting because they are advanced in age and are women, it does not mean that another will react the same way.

There is no doubt that intermittent fasting is not meant for everyone. Fasting is not safe for children because they need all the food they can get for continual development. Fasting in itself is not the issue for older people – any adult can fast.

Myth #2: You Gain Weight as You Age

A myth is a combination of facts and falsehood. This is a typical example of that. It is saying that growing older means your metabolism will slow down and your body will not burn or use up calories as fast as when you were younger. However, weight gain in older adults is not a given. The key to keeping your body performing optimally is to develop and maintain healthy habits such as fasting intermittently, drinking enough water, reducing stress levels, and getting adequate exercise.

Myth #3: Your Metabolism Slows Down During Fasting

This myth represents one of those big misunderstandings I mentioned earlier. The difference between calorie restriction and deliberately choosing when to take in calories is huge. Intermittent fasting does not necessarily limit calorie intake neither does it make you starve. It is when a person starves or under-eats that changes occur in their metabolic rate. But there is no change whatsoever in your metabolism when you delay eating for a few hours by fasting intermittently.

Myth #4: You Will Get Fat If You Skip Breakfast

"Breakfast is the most important meal of the day!" This is one of the more popular urban myths about intermittent fasting. It is in the same category with the myths, *"Santa doesn't give you presents if your naughty,"* and *"carrots give you night vision."* Some people will readily point to a relative or friend who is fat because they don't eat breakfast. But the question is: are they fat because they don't eat breakfast? Or do they skip breakfast because they are fat and want to reduce their calorie intake?

The best way to collect unbiased data when conducting scientific studies is through randomized controlled trials (RTC). After a careful study of 13 different RTCs on the relationship weight gain and eating or skipping breakfast, researchers from Melbourne, Australia found that both overweight and normal-weight participants who ate breakfast gained more weight than participants who skipped breakfast. The researchers also found that there's a higher rate of calorie consumption later in the day in participants who ate breakfast. This puts a hole in the popular notion that skipping breakfast will make people overeat later in the day (Harvard Medical School, 2019).

The truth is, there is nothing spectacular about eating breakfast as far as weight management is concerned. There is limited scientific evidence disproving or supporting the idea that breakfast influences weight. Instead, studies only show that there is no difference in weight loss or gain when one eats or skips breakfast.

Myth #5: Exercise Is Harmful to Older Adults Especially While Fasting

No. It is not harmful to exercise while fasting. And no, exercise is not harmful to older adults, whether they are fasting or not. On the contrary, exercising during your fasting window helps to burn stored fats in the body. When you perform physical activities after eating, your body tries to burn off new calories that are ingested from your meal. But when you exercise on an empty or nearly empty stomach, your body burns fats that are stored already and keeps you fit.

What is harmful to older adults is not engaging in exercises at all. A lack of exercise or adequate physical activity in older adults is linked to diabetes, heart disease, and obesity among other health conditions.

Researchers from Harvard Medical School demonstrated in a landmark study that frail and old women could regain functional loss through resistance exercise (Harvard Medical School, 2007). For ten weeks, participants from a nursing home (100 women aged between 72 and 98) performed resistance exercises three times a week. At the end of 10 weeks, the participants could walk faster, further, climb more stairs, and lift a great deal of weight than their inactive counterparts. Also, a 10-year study of healthy aging by researchers with the MacArthur Study of Aging in America found that older adults (people between 70 and 80 years) can get physically fit whether or not they have been exercising at their younger age. The bottom line is, as long as you can move the muscles in your body, do it because it is safe and will only help you live a better and longer life.

Myth #6: Eating Frequently Reduces Hunger

There is mixed scientific evidence in this regard. Some studies show that eating frequently reduces hunger in some people. On the other hand, other studies show the exact opposite. Interestingly, at least one study shows no difference in the frequency of eating and how it influences hunger (US National Library of Medicine, 2013). Eating can help some people get over cravings and excessive hunger, but there is no shred of evidence to prove that it applies to everyone.

Myth #7: "You Can't Teach an Old Dog New Tricks"

The brain never stops learning neither does it stop developing at any age. New neural pathways are created when a person learns something new at any age. And with continued repetition, the neural pathways become stronger until the behavior is habitual. Older people are often more persistent and have a higher motivation than younger people when it comes to learning new things. Learning should be a lifelong pursuit and not an activity reserved for young people.

Don't allow anyone to convince you into believing that it is too late to learn new eating habits because you are in your golden years or are approaching it. It doesn't matter if you've never tried fasting you can still train your brain to make fasting a habit even in old age. Start small, make it a natural occurrence in everyday life, repeating until you get used to it, and your positive results aka glowing skin, improved energy will motivate you to make it into a lifestyle.

Myth #8: You Must Lose Weight During Intermittent Fasting

This myth is rooted in the hype that intermittent fasting has received in recent years. Unless done correctly, intermittent fasting may not yield weight loss benefits. For you to experience any significant loss in weight, you must ensure that you eat healthily during your eating window. Equally, it is important to stick to the fasting schedule. If you keep cheating and adjusting your fasting window to favor more eating time or you overeat during the eating window to compensate for lost meals, your chances of losing weight will be greatly diminished.

Myth #9: Your Body Will Go Into "Starvation Mode" If You Practice Intermittent Fasting

This myth is based on the misconception of what the starvation mode is and what triggers it. First of all, starvation is when your body senses that there is a significant drop in energy supply and reduces your metabolic rate. In simple terms, it is a reduction in the rate at which your body burns fat as a lack of food. This is an automatic response to conserve energy. It makes sense to reduce energy consumption if there is little to no supply of further energy coming from meals. In other words, if you stay away from food for too long, your body activates the starvation mode and significantly stops any further loss of body fat.

Having said that, intermittent fasting does not trigger the starvation mode. Instead, intermittent fasting helps to increase your metabolic activities. Meaning, your body can burn more fat when you fast for short periods. Starvation mode is only triggered when you engage in prolonged fasting over 48 hours, a practice I do not recommend for older adults.

Myth #10: An Aging Skin Is Better Taken Care of With Anti-Aging Cream

This is not necessarily true. Brown spots, sagging skin, and wrinkles can indeed be reversed using expensive creams and topical treatments especially if a dermatologist prescribes them. These topical products exfoliate the top layer of your skin and make them appear smoother. However, that result (clear, smooth skin) is only a temporary effect.

A better way to look younger without any side effects is by activating autophagy. Engaging in mild stress-inducing activities such as intermittent fasting and exercising are the way. One key element to maintaining healthy skin is quenching your skin's thirst. Not drinking enough water can damage skin causing it to become dry, blemished, and lead to wrinkles. Drinking adequate amounts of water every day is the best approach to successfully "take the years off."

Myth #11: Fasting Deprives Your Brain of Adequate Dietary Glucose

Some people believe that your brain will underperform if you don't eat foods rich in carbohydrates. This myth is rooted in the notion that your brain uses only glucose as its fuel. But your brain doesn't use only dietary glucose for fuel. Some very low-carb diets can cause your body to produce ketone bodies from high-fat foods. Your brain can function well on ketone bodies. Continuous, intermittent fasting coupled with exercise can trigger the production of ketone bodies. Additionally, your body can also use a process known as gluconeogenesis to produce the sugar needed by your brain. This means that your body can effectively produce it on its own without you feeding it with just carbs.

Intermittent fasting does not interfere with brain function or its fuel or energy needs. However, because intermittent fasting is not suitable for everyone, if you feel shaky, dizzy, or extremely fatigued during fasting, consider talking with your doctor or reducing your fasting window.

Myth #12: Intermittent Fasting Will Make Older Adults Lose Their Muscle

First of all, it is stereotypical and largely incorrect to think of older people as frail. Frailty is not limited to just older adults and is a generalization of old age. Younger people can become frail if they suffer from a disabling chronic disease or have a poor diet. Scientists studied data from almost half a million people and found that middle-aged adults as young as 37 show signs of frailty (Mail Online, 2018).

Secondly, intermittent fasting does not lead to muscle loss, whether in young or older people. On the contrary, fasting intermittently can help you maintain better muscle mass. It is, therefore, not surprising that intermittent fasting is a common practice among bodybuilders to help them maintain muscle mass.

Myth #13: All Fasting Outcomes Are The Same

This myth is rooted in the assumption that everyone has exactly the same physical and chemical makeup. No two individuals are the same regardless of how identical they appear to be. Age, existing medical conditions, body types and size, level of commitment to the practice are among the many factors that can significantly influence your results.

A woman who fasts for twelve hours twice a week is likely to have a different result from another woman who fasts for 16 hours four times a week. Even when people follow the same fasting regimen, their results will still vary and that is to be expected. Fasting results are not typical in any way. Thinking something else can lead to a weird frame of mind full of unnecessary comparison, pushing yourself too hard, or giving up too soon because your results don't look anything like that of women you've seen.

Common Questions

To help you avoid common fasting mistakes, here are quick answers to some of the frequent questions people have about intermittent fasting.

Q. "Do I need to avoid calories outside meal times or just actual food?"

A. Regardless of the internet hype, there is no reputable scientific studies to show that certain foods are "negative-calorie" foods or completely calorie-free. If you must fast, avoid all foods and calorie-containing drinks during the eating period.

Q. "I don't consciously follow a fasting regimen but I eat only once a day with snacks and sweetened drinks. Is it possible to achieve the benefits of fasting even though I'm not religiously following the practice?"

A. If you are already used to eating only once a day, it should be a lot easier to adopt a fasting regimen and stick to it. But if you snack or consume high or empty calorie-containing drinks outside meal times you'll sabotage any benefits of fasting and forgo all efforts.

Q. "I drink coffee with cream and sugar every morning, as I don't like the taste of black coffee and it helps me get through my day. How do I blend my morning 'coffee ritual' with intermittent fasting?"

A. Whether it is coffee or any other foods you like to eat, you don't have to deprive yourself. All you need to do is adjust your fasting schedule to suit your long-established eating habit, provided it is a healthy one. Instead of fussing over what foods you'll be missing or not, break your fast when you have your morning coffee. For example, if you intend to fast for 14 hours daily and eat for the remaining 10, you could have your coffee with cream and sugar by 8 am and eat your last meal for the day by 6 pm. You don't have to delay or skip breakfast if it doesn't suit you.

Q. "I've been practicing intermittent fasting on and off for about 3 weeks and I still feel very hungry, tired, and weak. My body is not just adapting to the practice. Is this really for me?"

A. It is advisable to start the practice with a larger eating window to ease the transition, and then gradually increase the fasting time frame. If you start with a fasting regimen that is too dramatic, your body might find it difficult to adjust as quickly as you want. However, if you have taken the necessary precautions and still not adjusting to the eating pattern, it is best to seek expert medical advice.

Q. "How long do I have to wait after quitting a diet program to start intermittent fasting? Are there any negative side effects of starting intermittent fasting immediately after following a diet program?"

A. Unless under medical advisement, you can begin intermittent fasting as soon as you think is comfortable for you. Only keep in mind that it is important not to cut back on your calorie intake as many diet programs suggest.

Q. "When does the fasting window start counting? For example, if my last meal for the day starts by 7 pm and ends at 8 pm, do I start counting my fasting window from 7 pm or 8 pm?

A. Your fast commences when you stop eating your last meal for the day. In the example above, the fast starts as soon as you finish your meal by 8 pm or at any time you finish your last meal.

Bottom Line

A lot of incorrect information is perpetuated about meal frequency and intermittent fasting. Many of the information are false, misconceptions, pure myth, and some are just outright insane.

Intermittent fasting may not be suitable for everyone, but it shouldn't be considered unhealthy as it offers tremendous health benefits. Hopefully, this book has cleared some of your misgivings and doubts about intermittent fasting. But if you are still unsure about any information regarding intermittent fasting, especially as it affects you in particular, I strongly suggest that you speak with your doctor.

Conclusion

Women have a tendency to be more reactionary, cautionary, and emotional than men. That means you are more likely to start applying the things you've learned in this book and have it make a difference in your life than the average man if he were to read a similar book.

Before you jump in, I suggest you take the time to do more research, and really take into consideration what you've read and then ask yourself why you want to do this in the first place. Once you've discovered strong reasons to anchor your actions, it will be easier to move forward when you are faced with difficulties down the road. Because there is no sugar-coating it, you will face some rough patches where you will want to quit. But you are a strong-willed goddess! That is the advantage of learning as an older adult. What most young people will face, struggle with and ultimately throw in the towel, you will gleefully excel at by drawing on your wealth of experience to overcome any hurdle.

Although I have written this book for all older women, it would be a classic mistake to put you all in one category. You are a unique individual, therefore, approach the suggestions and recommendations in this book as a guideline with flexibility that can be mended to suit you the best. This book was written to give you a broad perspective on intermittent fasting. It is now your turn to dip your toe in the water, so to speak, and try these various methods as a test. When you find the method that resonates with you and suits your specific needs, commit to it. With time, you will master the method and even introduce a few changes to make it your customized intermittent fasting plan.

It is the norm for people to try out intermittent fasting as a solution for various health problems. However, to get the most out of the practice, it is better to approach it as a new way of life. That is to say, even after achieving your health goal (weight loss, improved cognitive function, balanced hormones, healthier skin), you should continue practicing intermittent fasting as a regular part of your day. Don't throw it all away because you've reached a few milestones. Remember that one of the benefits of fasting intermittently is to increase longevity. While you may not normally follow a rigorous diet plan as you would in the early stages of fasting, you do need to maintain these habits to keep reaping its benefits.

When you are in great shape, you will have things to look forward to as any healthy woman should, regardless of her age. The life expectancy of women is on the rise so why endure a poor quality of life for even longer? Never buy into the ideas that your body has to decline with age. Don't just allow life to change, make it change for you!

Made in the USA
Las Vegas, NV
19 October 2022

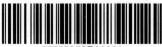

57755858R00061